Pocket

Infectious Diseases
Second Edition

Withdrawn

W. Edmund Farrar MD, FACP
Professor of Medicine and Microbiology
Medical University of South Carolina
Charleston, South Carolina, USA

Martin J. Wood FRCP
Consultant Physician
East Birmingham Hospital
Birmingham, UK

John A. Innes BSc, FRCP, FRCP (Ed.)
Consultant Physician
East Birmingham Hospital
Birmingham, UK

Hugh Tubbs MBBS, MRCS, MSc, DCH, FRCP
Consultant Physician and Senior Lecturer
North Staffordshire Hospital Centre
Stoke-on-Trent, UK

Gower Medical Publishing • London • New York

Distributed in the USA and Canada by:

Raven Press Ltd
1185 Avenue of the Americas
New York
New York 10036
USA

Distributed in the rest of the world by:

Gower Medical Publishing
Middlesex House
34–42 Cleveland Street
London W1P 5FB
UK

Cataloguing in Publication Data:

Catalogue records for this book are available from the US Library of Congress and British Library.

ISBN 1–56375–533–5

Project manager:	Stephen McGrath
Design:	Ian Spick
Index:	Nina Boyd
Production	Susan Bishop
Publisher	Fiona Foley

Typesetting on Apple Macintosh®.
CRC output by The Text Unit.
Text set in New Century Schoolbook; captions set in Helvetica.
Originated in Hong Kong by Bright Arts (HK) Ltd.
Printed in Hong Kong.
Produced by Imago Services (HK) Ltd.

PREFACE

In this book we have collected 171 pictures to illustrate a wide variety of infectious diseases. Most of these conditions are common in one or another part of the world, but we have also included some less familiar diseases which present characteristic appearances and have important therapeutic implications.

Most of the pictures are clinical photographs, but radiographs and microscopic appearances of clinical specimens and pathogenic microorgansims are also included. We hope that this collection will provide a valuable and useful guide for both clinicians and laboratory workers.

A more comprehensive account of infectious diseases, including more than 1300 photographs and line drawings, is available in *Infectious Diseases: Text and Color Atlas*, by the same authors.

WEF
MJW
JAI
HT

Charleston, Birmingham and Stoke-on-Trent, 1992.

CONTENTS

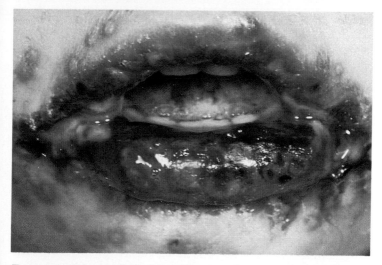

Fig. 1 Herpes simplex virus infection. Vesicular lesions on the skin of the upper and lower lips and cheeks of a child with primary infection. Gingivostomatitis is the commonest manifestation of primary infection with herpes simplex virus type I. Vesicular lesions may appear on the tongue, gingiva, buccal mucosa, lips and surrounding skin; these later rupture to form painful, shallow ulcers.

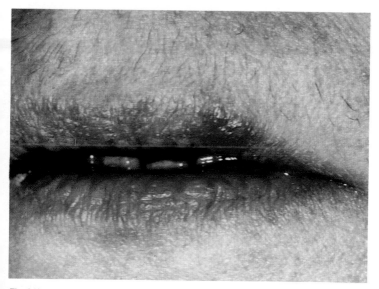

Fig. 2 Herpes simplex virus infection. Vesicular lesions ('fever blisters') on the mucocutaneous junction of the lip. This is the typical location of recurrent disease; typically only a few lesions are present.

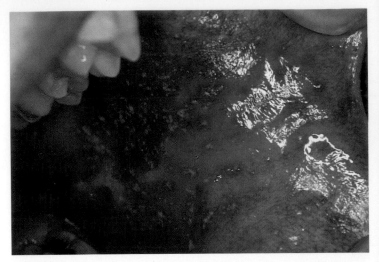

Fig. 3 Measles. Koplik's spots on the buccal mucosa. These tiny white lesions, which resemble damp grains of salt on the mucosa opposite the premolar teeth, are highly specific for measles and often precede the development of the rash, allowing an early diagnosis to be made.

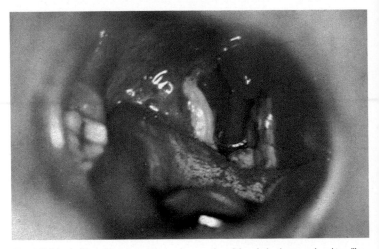

Fig. 4 Diphtheria. There is gross swelling and congestion of the whole pharyngeal and tonsillar area. A dirty white exudate covers the tonsils and is spreading to the posterior pharyngeal wall. There is often local lymph node enlargement and oedema of the subcutaneous tissues ('bull neck'). Presence of diphtheritic membranes in the larynx or trachea may cause obstruction of the airway. Courtesy of Dr K. Nye.

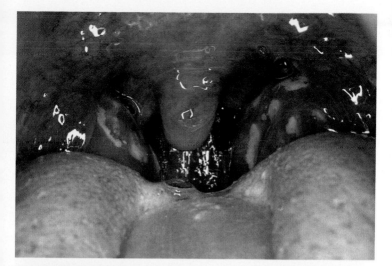

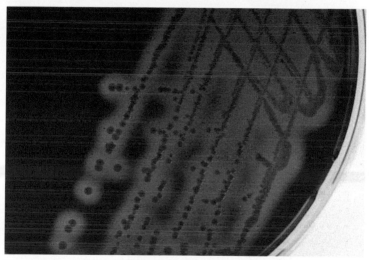

Fig. 5 Streptococcal tonsillitis. Top: There is intense erythema of the tonsils and surrounding tissue, with a creamy yellow exudate. Bottom: The diagnosis can be made with certainty only by identifying *Streptococcus pyogenes* in a culture from the throat. On a blood agar plate the bacterial colonies are surrounded by a clear zone of β-haemolysis.

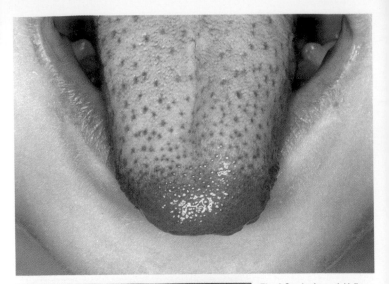

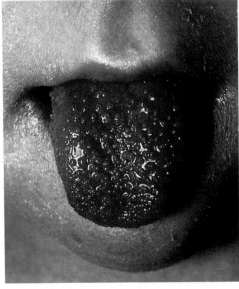

Fig. 6 Scarlet fever. Initially the tongue is covered by a white exudate through which the papillae project (white strawberry tongue – above). Later the exudate is shed to reveal the bright red inflammation of the underlying tissue (red strawberry tongue – left).

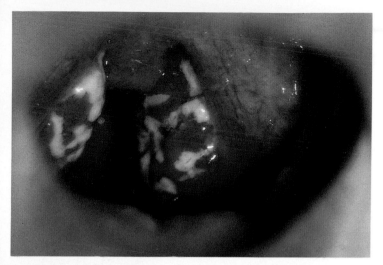

Fig. 7 Infectious mononucleosis. There is gross tonsillar enlargement with a white exudate. The appearance may resemble streptococcal pharyngitis, but in infectious mononucleosis there is often generalized lymphadenopathy, splenomegaly, hepatitis and atypical lymphocytes in the peripheral blood.

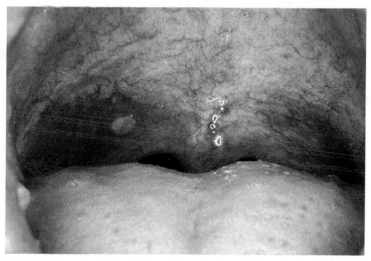

Fig. 8 Pharyngoconjunctival fever. Lesions of the palate due to infection with adenovirus type 3. The painful ulcerative lesions in the mouth are often accompanied by follicular conjunctivitis. Somewhat similar oral lesions may be seen in herpangina and hand, foot and mouth disease, illnesses caused by Coxsackie A viruses.

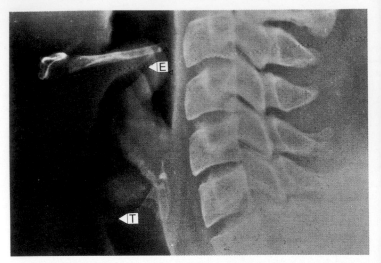

Fig. 9 Acute epiglottitis. Lateral radiograph of the neck showing the tracheal air shadow (T) and rounded swollen tissue shadow of the enlarged epiglottis (E). This dangerous infection, most often seen in young children and almost always caused by *Haemophilus influenzae* type b, can cause sudden obstruction of the airway and may require emergency tracheotomy and antibiotic therapy.

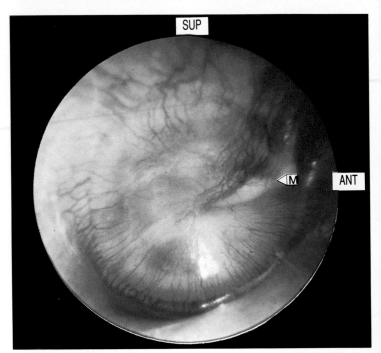

Fig. 10 Acute otitis media. Early stage showing mild injection of the drum, especially in the region of the malleus (M). The most common bacterial causes are *Streptococcus pneumoniae* and *Haemophilus influenzae*, with a smaller proportion of cases caused by *Streptococcus pyogenes* or *Branhamella catarrhalis*. Courtesy of Dr M. Chaput de Saintonge.

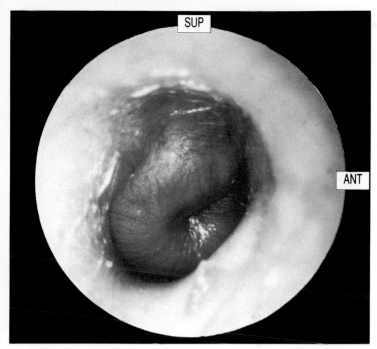

Fig. 11 Acute otitis media. Advanced stage showing bulging of the drum on both sides of the malleus, which is obscured. These features are seen just before the drum perforates. By courtesy of Dr M. Chaput de Saintonge.

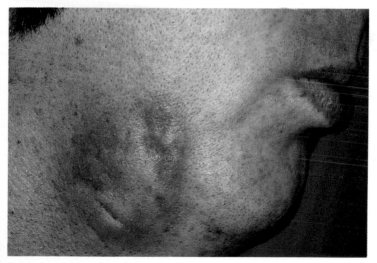

Fig. 12 Actinomycosis. The cervicofacial form is most common, arising from a dental infection. There is erythema and induration of the overlying skin, and a chronic draining sinus may be present. By courtesy of Mr C. J. Meryon.

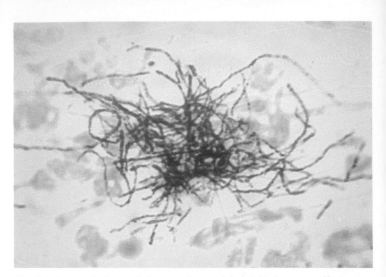

Fig. 13 Actinomycosis. Gram stain from an actinomycotic lesion showing gram-positive branching filaments of *Actinomyces israelii*. These yellow-coloured gritty clumps of organisms and inflammatory cells may be seen with the naked eye or low power microscope and are known as 'sulphur granules'. By courtesy of Ms A. E. Prevost.

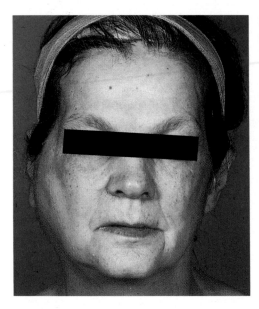

Fig. 14 Acute bacterial parotitis. This infection, usually caused by *Staphylococcus aureus*, is seen most commonly in debilitated individuals who breathe through the mouth. There is enlargement of the parotid gland with extreme tenderness and erythema of the overlying skin.

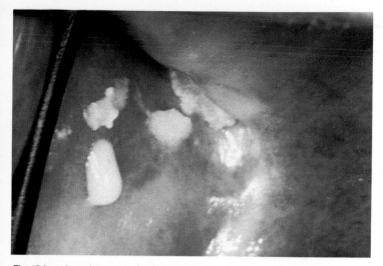

Fig. 15 Acute bacterial parotitis. Gentle pressure on the gland may cause extrusion of creamy pus from the orifice of Stensen's duct.

LOWER RESPIRATORY TRACT

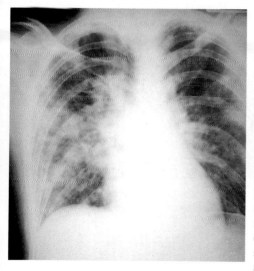

Fig. 16 Varicella pneumonia. Chest radiograph showing widespread patchy infiltrates throughout both lungs in a patient with Hodgkin's disease. This disease is occasionally seen in children with chickenpox. In adults it usually occurs in immunocompromised individuals, often causing a life-threatening illness. Pneumonia may be caused by many viruses, including measles virus, cytomegalovirus, herpes simplex virus, influenza virus and all of the viruses which cause acute bronchitis.

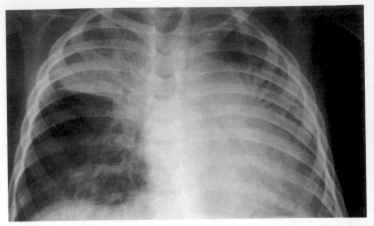

Fig. 17 Pneumococcal pneumonia. Chest radiograph showing lobar consolidation affecting both lungs. An air bronchogram is easily seen in the left middle zone. *Streptococcus pneumoniae* is the commonest cause of community-acquired pneumonia in previously healthy individuals. The characteristic pattern is a lobar consolidation, but bronchopneumonia and segmental areas of consolidation are also seen.

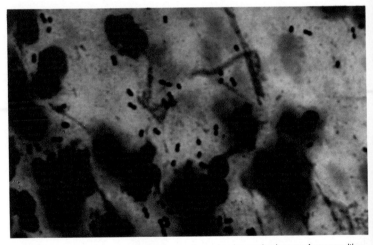

Fig. 18 Pneumococcal pneumonia. Sputum specimen showing predominance of gram-positive lancet-shaped diplococci. Gram's stain. Courtesy of Dr J. R. Cantey.

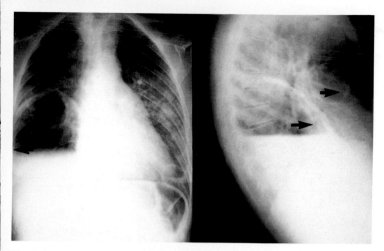

Fig. 19 Staphylococcal pneumonia. Posteroanterior and lateral chest radiographs of an infant showing pneumatoceles (arrowed) in the right middle and lower lobes and in the left lower lobe. These thin-walled cavities often heal rapidly and completely. In adults staphylococcal pneumonia often occurs as a complication of influenza virus infection.

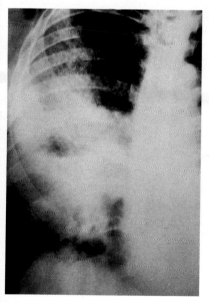

Fig. 20 Klebsiella pneumonia. Chest radiograph showing extensive consolidation in the right lung with a central area of necrosis and abscess formation. Cavitation is a common feature of pneumonia due to *Klebsiella* and other gram-negative bacilli.

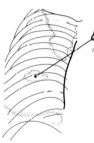

cavity within consolidated area

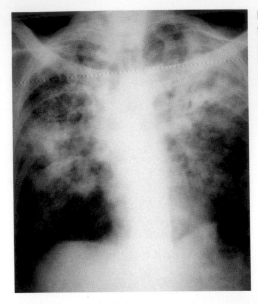

Fig. 21 Pulmonary tuberculosis. Chest radiograph showing extensive bilateral infiltrates most prominent in the upper lobes, with areas of cavitation. This picture is characteristic of far advanced disease.

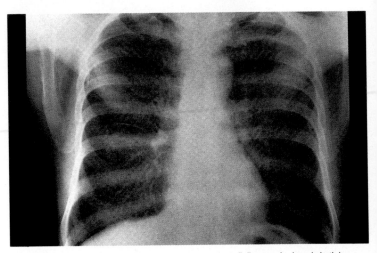

Fig. 22 Tuberculosis. This x-ray shows very widespread small discrete shadows in both lung fields. The patient has miliary tuberculosis, a sequel of haematogenous dissemination of the organism which may develop in the post-primary phase or in patients with long-standing latent infection. Miliary tuberculosis is also encountered in patients with immunosuppression.

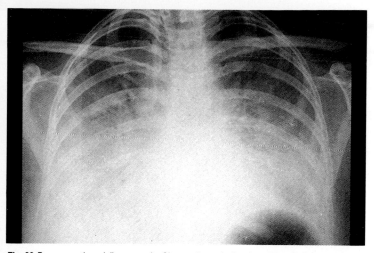

Fig. 23 *Pneumocystis carinii* pneumonia. Chest radiograph showing advanced disease with dense infiltrates in both lungs. This disease is extremely common in patients with AIDS, but is also observed in severe malnutrition and other types of immunosuppression. Severe hypoxaemia is often present. This film shows the classic appearance with symmetrical 'ground-glass' opacities in both lower lung fields, but the radiographic and clinical features are highly variable.

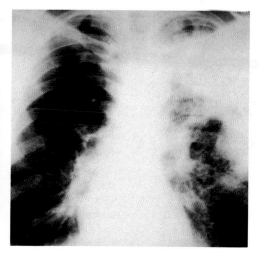

Fig. 24 Chronic histoplasmosis. Radiograph showing contraction of left upper lobe with multiple cavities. The self-limited pneumonitis of acute histoplasmosis is non-specific, but the disease may progress to a chronic pneumonia which resembles tuberculosis, as in this case.

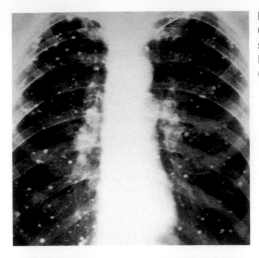

Fig. 25 Histoplasmosis. Chest radiograph showing scattered calcification in healed miliary lesions. Courtesy of Dr M. Pearson.

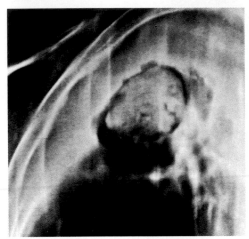

Fig. 26 Aspergilloma. Tomogram of lung cavity containing fungus ball outlined by air space. This lesion, which usually involves a pre-existing cavity in the lung, is occasionally associated with haemoptysis.

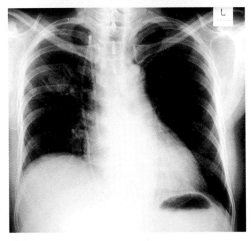

Fig. 27 Invasive aspergillosis. Chest radiograph showing early lesion in the right lung of a neutropenic patient with acute myeloblastic leukaemia. This disease, seen in severely immunocompromised patients, is usually fatal unless treatment is initiated promptly with amphotericin B.

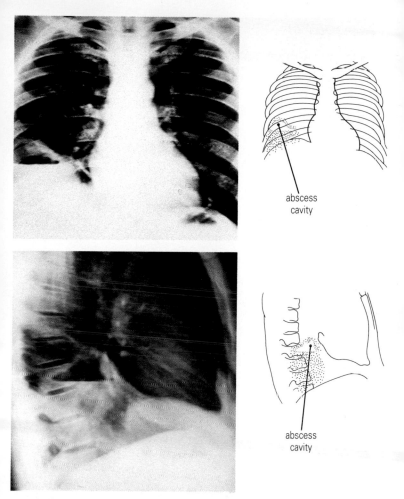

Fig. 28 Aspiration lung abscess. Chest radiographs, posteroanterior and lateral, showing abscess cavity in lower lobe of right lung. This disease results from aspiration of secretions and bacteria from the upper respiratory tract.

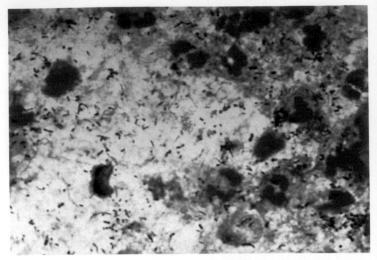

Fig. 29 Aspiration lung abscess. Sample of pus showing abundant microorganisms, including gram-positive cocci and various gram-negative and gram-positive rods. Gram's stain. Courtesy of Dr J. R. Cantey.

THE NERVOUS SYSTEM

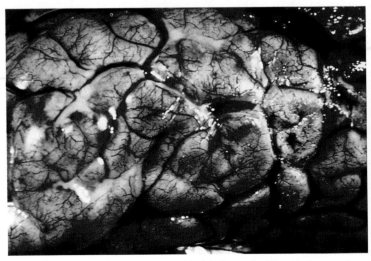

Fig. 30 Bacterial meningitis. Gross specimen of fresh brain revealing intense acute congestion of meningeal blood vessels and purulent exudate in sulci. The most common causes of bacterial meningitis outside the neonatal period are *Streptococcus pneumoniae*, *Neisseria meningitidis* and *Haemophilus influenzae*, all of which inhabit the mucosal surface of the nasopharynx.

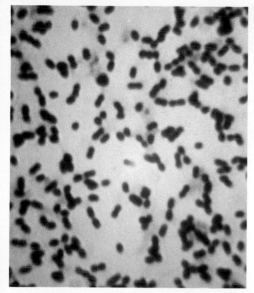

Fig. 31 Pneumococcal meningitis. Large numbers of gram-positive diplococci in cerebrospinal fluid with only a few fragments of degenerating polymorphonuclear leucocytes. This pattern of abundant bacteria with few or no phagocytic cells in the CSF is associated with a poor prognosis for survival. Gram's stain. Courtesy of Dr T. F. Sellers, Jr.

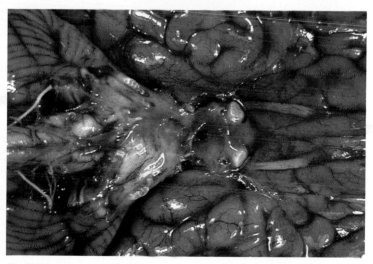

Fig. 32 Tuberculous meningitis. Autopsy specimen of fresh brain showing the thickened gelatinous basal meninges, especially thick in the region of the optic chiasma and over the pons. The chronic basilar meningitis often causes dysfunction of various cranial nerves.

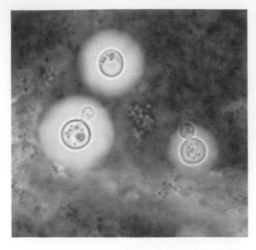

Fig. 33 Cryptococcal meningitis. Stained CSF sediment demonstrating the prominent capsule of the organism. Note the highly refractile cell wall and internal structure of the yeast. India ink preparation. Courtesy of Ms A. E. Prevost.

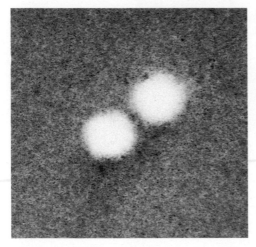

Fig. 34 Lymphocytes in CSF sediment. Note that these cells lack the prominent refractile cell wall and internal structure seen in *Cryptococcus neoformans*. India ink preparation. Courtesy of Dr J. R. Cantey.

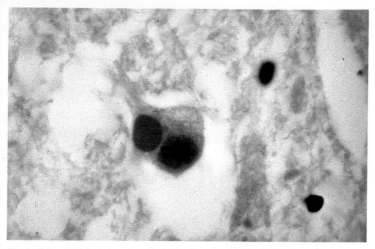

Fig. 35 Rabies. Histological section of brain showing a Negri body. (H&E stain.) These eosinophilic cytoplasmic inclusions, which often contain basophilic spots, are found in 70–80% of cases, most commonly in the hippocampus. They may be demonstrated by conventional histological techniques or by immunofluorescent staining.

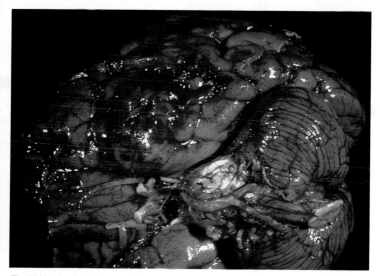

Fig. 36 Herpes simplex encephalitis. Gross specimen of brain showing necrosis, haemorrhage and oedema involving the orbital surface of the left frontal lobe and the anterior, medial and lateral surfaces of the left temporal lobe. These are characteristic locations of the lesions in this disease.

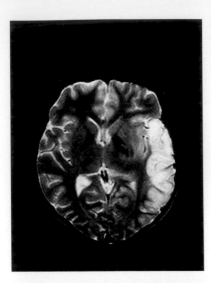

Fig. 37 Herpes simplex encephalitis. MRI scan showing extensive involvement of the left temporal area. Courtesy of Dr J. Curé.

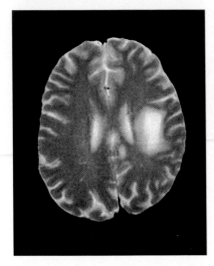

Fig. 38 Progressive multifocal leucoencephalopathy. MRI scan showing a large lesion in the left parietal region and a smaller lesion closer to the midline. This demyelinating disease, due to a polyomavirus, is an uncommon opportunistic infection in patients with AIDS and other immunosuppressing conditions. It usually progresses to death within a few months of onset. Courtesy of Dr J. Curé.

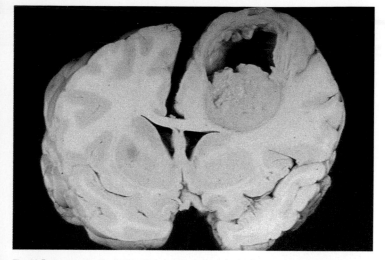

Fig. 39 Brain abscess. Coronal section revealing chronic brain abscess due to *Staphylococcus aureus* in the left frontal lobe of a 16-year-old girl. The border of the abscess cavity reveals a linear region of brownish discolouration which represents the capsule of the abscess.

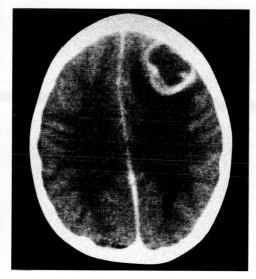

Fig. 40 Brain abscess. CT scan showing the typical appearance of a brain abscess in the left frontal lobe with enhancement of the capsule. The uniform thin wall is characteristic of abscess rather than tumour. Courtesy of Dr G. D. Hungerford.

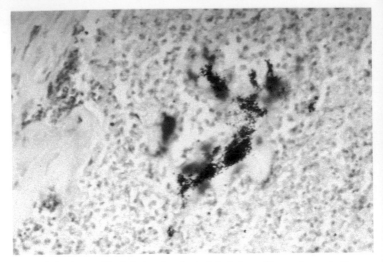

Fig. 41 Brain abscess. Histological section of necrotic brain tissue. Clumps of gram-positive bacteria can be seen within the necrotic material. Brown and Brenn stain. Courtesy of Dr J. R. Cantey.

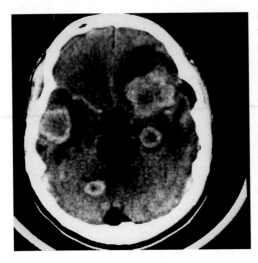

Fig. 42 Cerebral toxoplasmosis. CT scan showing multiple ring-enhancing hypodense lesions, in the left frontotemporal, right temporal, right occipital and left uncal regions, with surrounding cerebral oedema. Toxoplasma encephalitis is the most common opportunistic infection of the central nervous system in patients with AIDS.

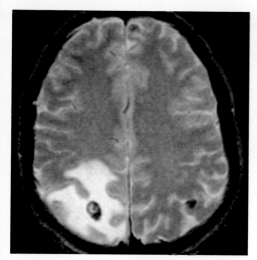

Fig. 43 Cerebral cysticercosis. MRI scan showing a cyst containing a developing larva, surrounded by an area of oedema. The disease may present with headache, papilloedema, focal neurological signs and seizures. Praziquantel is effective in killing the larval stage of the organism. Courtesy of Dr J. Curé.

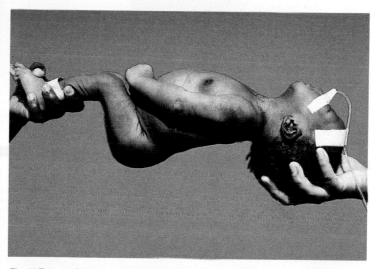

Fig. 44 Tetanus. Opisthotonus in an infant due to intense contraction of the paravertebral muscles. Neonatal tetanus occurs primarily in developing countries, and is often related to contamination of the umbilical stump. Courtesy of Dr T. F. Sellers, Jr.

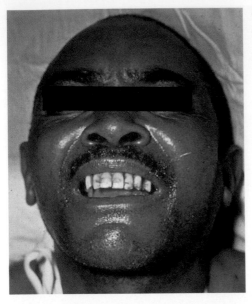

Fig. 45 Tetanus. Risus sardonicus, the 'sardonic smile', due to spasm of the facial muscles. Courtesy of Dr T. F. Sellers, Jr.

THE GASTROINTESTINAL TRACT

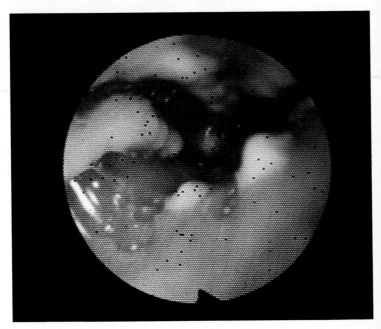

Fig. 46 Candida oesophagitis. Severe oesophagitis with ulceration, showing discrete ulcers and thrushlike plaques on the mucosa. This is a common opportunistic infection in patients with AIDS. Courtesy of Dr J. Cunningham.

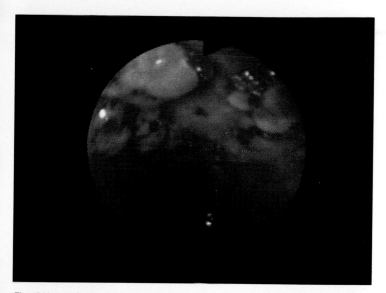

Fig. 47 Herpes simplex oesophagitis. Endoscopic view showing herpetic vesicles and multiple ulcers. Like candida oesophagitis, this disease is seen primarily in individuals with AIDS or other immunosuppressing conditions.

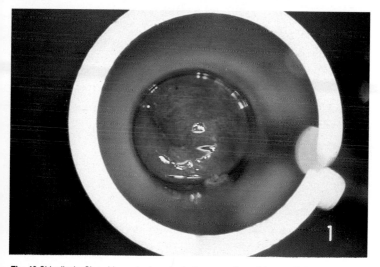

Fig. 48 Shigellosis. Sigmoidoscopic view of colonic mucosa in a mild case of infection due to *Shigella flexneri*. Note the thin whitish exudate, which is made up of fibrin and polymorphonuclear leucocytes. This type of non-specific colitis may be seen in other enteric infections due to invasive bacteria. Courtesy of Dr R. H. Gilman.

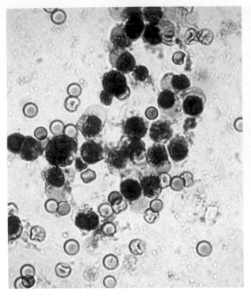

Fig. 49 Shigellosis. Polymorphonuclear and mononuclear leucocytes and red blood cells in the stool of a patient with shigellosis. Presence of inflammatory cells in faeces is characteristic of infections due to invasive microorganisms. Methylene blue wet mount under cover slip. Courtesy of Dr H. L. DuPont.

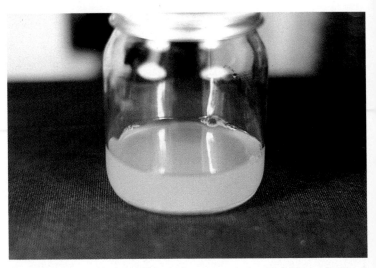

Fig. 50 Rice water stool in cholera. The voluminous watery stool excreted at the height of the illness is nearly colourless and contains flecks of mucus. Effects of the disease can be reversed by replacement of water and electrolyte losses. Courtesy of Dr A. M. Geddes.

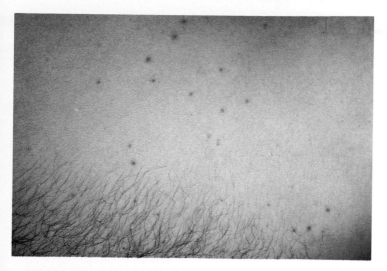

Fig. 51 Typhoid fever. Rose spots, small maculopapular erythematous lesions usually seen on the abdomen. Courtesy of Dr A. M. Geddes.

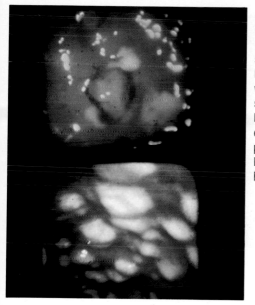

Fig. 52 Antibiotic-associated colitis due to *Clostridium difficile*. Colonoscopic views showing the characteristic lesions. Upper: Several whitish or yellowish plaques surrounded by haemorrhagic borders. Lower: Numerous characteristic whitish placques. Courtesy of Dr F. Pittman (upper) and Dr R. Fekety (lower).

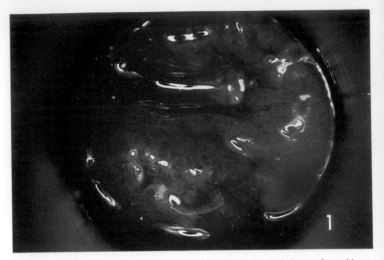

Fig. 53 Amoebic colitis. Sigmoidoscopic view of colonic mucosa in a typical case of amoebic dysentery, showing the non-ulcerated diffuse colitis which is the predominant form of the disease. Courtesy of Dr R. H. Gilman.

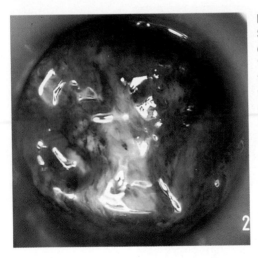

Fig. 54 Amoebic colitis. Sigmoidoscopic view of colonic mucosa showing the 'textbook', but less common form of amoebic dysentery, with deep ulcers and overlying purulent exudate. By courtesy of Dr R. H. Gilman.

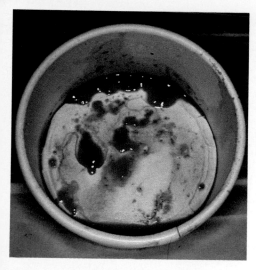

Fig. 55 Amoebic colitis. Typical dysentery stool (small volume, blood, pus and mucus) from a patient with acute amoebiasis. This type of stool is also seen in other infections in which there is microbial invasion of the bowel wall. Courtesy of Dr H. L. DuPont.

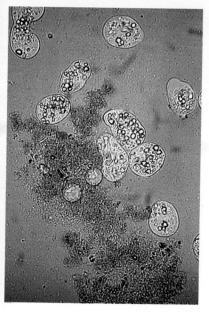

Fig. 56 Amoebic colitis. Trophozoites of *Entamoeba histolytica* showing amoeboid form and internal organelles. Motile trophozoites can often be found in acute amoebic colitis by examining a fleck of mucus from a fresh stool specimen on a warm microscope stage. Eosin stain.

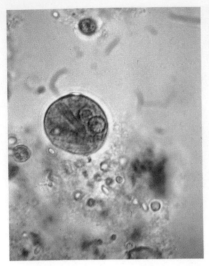

Fig. 57 Amoebic colitis. Cyst of *Entamoeba histolytica* showing round shape, refractile wall and multiple nuclei. Iodine stain.

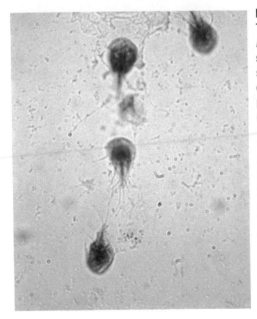

Fig. 58 Giardiasis. Trophozoites of *Giardia lamblia* obtained from mucus stripped from an Enterotest string pulled from the duodenum after overnight passage. Note the characteristic shape, paired nuclei and multiple flagella. The patient also had adult-acquired hypogammaglobulinaemia. Three stool examinations for *G. lamblia* had been negative. Trichrome stain. By courtesy of Dr F. Pittman.

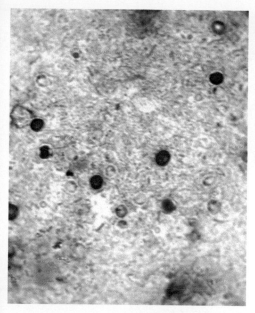

Fig. 59 Cryptosporidiosis. Modified acid-fast stain of stool specimen showing characteristic acid-fast cryptosporidium organisms. This infection, which is usually benign in immunocompetent individuals, may produce a relentless, progressive diarrhoeal illness in patients with AIDS.

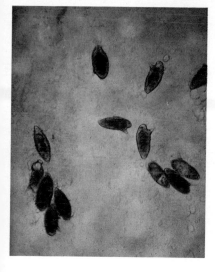

Fig. 60 Schistosomiasis. Eggs of *Schistosoma mansoni* in faeces showing the characteristic lateral spine. The three species of schistosomes important in human disease infect more than 200 million people worldwide.

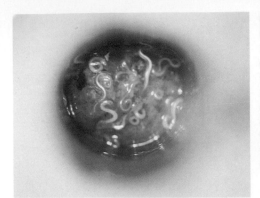

Fig. 61 Trichuriasis. Numerous adult *Trichuris trichiura* seen on proctoscopic examination in a healthy infected child. The thin anterior 'whip' end of the worm is secured within the intestinal mucosa and the thicker posterior end is seen within the lumen. Courtesy of Dr R. H. Gilman.

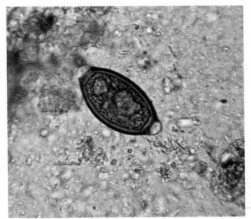

Fig. 62 Trichuriasis. Egg of *Trichuris trichiura* in faeces. Note the barrel-shaped, thick shell and translucent polar prominences.

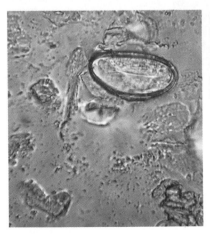

Fig. 63 Enterobiasis (pinworm or threadworm infection). A characteristic egg of *Enterobius vermicularis*, collected by adhesive cellophane tape pressed against the perianal area early in the morning.

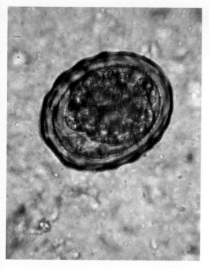

Fig. 64 Ascariasis. Embryonated egg of *Ascaris lumbricoides* containing a mature embryo and exhibiting relatively little cortication of the outer shell.

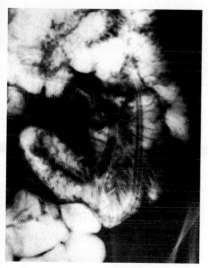

Fig. 65 Ascariasis. Barium study of small bowel in a patient with ascariasis. The intestinal tract of one of the adult worms is also well outlined with barium which it has ingested.

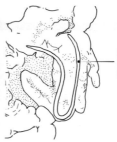

adult worm in small bowel

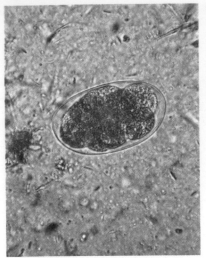

Fig. 66 Hookworm infection. Embryonated egg of *Necator americanus* in which cell division has begun. In freshly passed stool specimens the eggs seen are non-embryonated, but if the specimen has been at room temperature for several hours, embryos of various stages may be seen within the eggs.

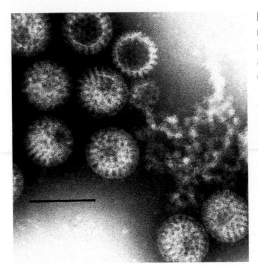

Fig. 67 Rotavirus. Electron micrograph showing negatively-stained particles, approximately 75 nm in diameter, in faeces. The 'spoked wheel' appearance is characteristic. (Bar = 100 nm.) Rotaviruses are often present in such large amounts in diarrhoeal stools that they can be identified directly by electron microscopy. Rotaviruses are the most important viral causes of diarrhoea worldwide; they produce a relatively prolonged illness which may result in severe dehydration in small children.

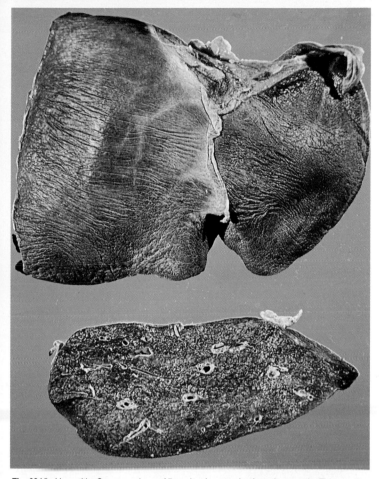

Fig. 68 Viral hepatitis. Gross specimen of liver showing massive hepatic necrosis. The capsular surface (upper) is wrinkled. The cut surface (lower) has a 'nutmeg' appearance due to cell loss and congestion in the central lobular zones. Light foci represent remaining liver cells; areas of necrosis appear darker. The hepatic architecture has collapsed and the organ has shrunk in size. This type of fulminant hepatitis with hepatic failure and encephalopathy occurs occasionally in hepatitis B infection. It is often associated with mutant forms of the hepatitis B virus or with concomitant infection with hepatitis delta virus. Courtesy of Dr J. Newman.

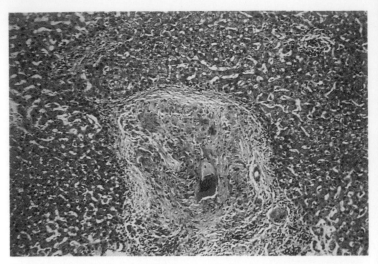

Fig. 69 Schistosomiasis. Eggs of *Schistosoma mansoni* in liver with surrounding granulomatous reaction. H&E stain. If the number of schistosomes in the liver is very large, portal hypertension, hepatosplenomegaly and oesophageal varices may result.

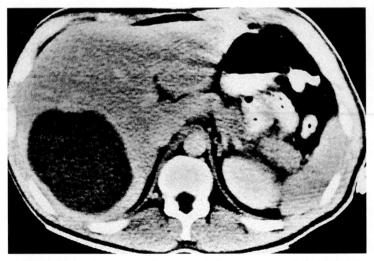

Fig. 70 Amoebic liver abscess. Scan showing large single amoebic abscess in the right lobe of the liver. Most patients do not give a history consistent with preceding or current amoebic dysentery. The serological test for amoebiasis is almost always positive. Courtesy of Dr F. Pittman.

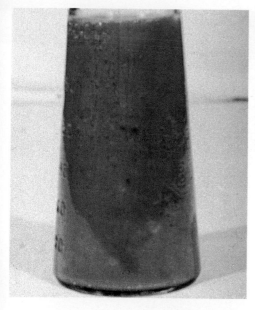

Fig. 71 Amoebic liver abscess. 'Anchovy paste' material aspirated from an amoebic abscess of the liver. This fluid, unlike that found in pyogenic liver abscess, is odourless. Amoebae may or may not be readily found upon microscopic examination. Courtesy of Dr K. Juniper.

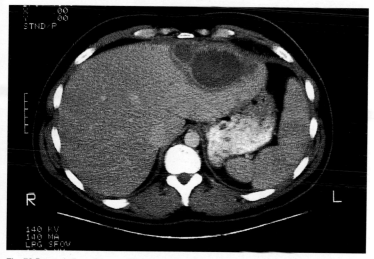

Fig. 72 Pyogenic liver abscess. CT scan showing a large abscess in the left lobe of the liver, with septum formation between compartments of the abscess. Bacterial abscesses of the liver are often multiple, and the patient may be severely ill with high fever and shaking chills. Courtesy of Dr R. Noble.

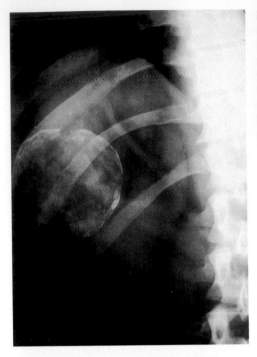

Fig. 73 Echinococcosis. Abdominal radiograph showing a calcified hydatid cyst in the liver. The liver and the lung are the most common sites for hydatid cysts. Serological tests often provide a specific aetiological diagnosis.

THE URINARY TRACT

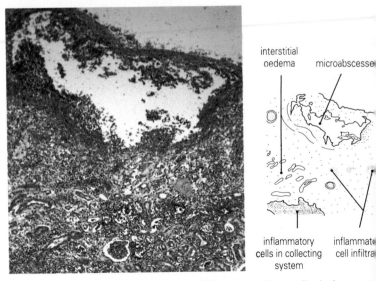

interstitial oedema   microabscesse

inflammatory cells in collecting system   inflammate cell infiltra

Fig. 74 Acute pyelonephritis. Histological section of kidney showing intense infiltration by inflammatory cells, severe interstitial oedema, many inflammatory cells in the collecting system and an intrarenal abscess. H&E stain.

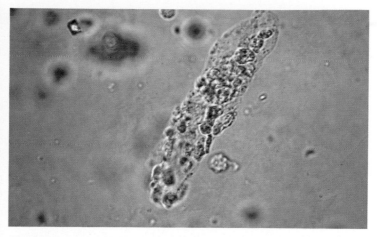

Fig. 75 Acute pyelonephritis. High power view of urine sediment showing a tubular cast containing many white blood cells in various stages of degeneration. These casts containing white blood cells are formed in the renal tubules and collecting ducts and thus signify involvement of the kidney. Courtesy of Dr S. Rous.

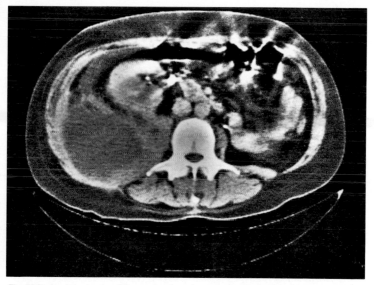

Fig. 76 Perinephric abscess. CT scan showing a large abscess in the right perinephric space, with marked anterior displacement of the right kidney. CT scanning and ultrasound studies have greatly aided in the diagnosis of this condition. Courtesy of Dr P. Hohl.

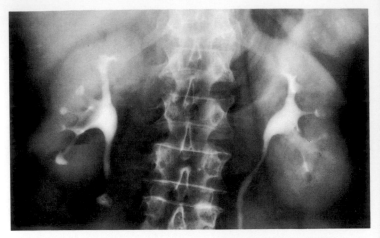

Fig. 77 Chronic pyelonephritis. Intravenous urogram at 15 minutes showing asymmetric contraction and distortion of the outline of the right kidney, with deep cortical scarring opposite blunted calices. Courtesy of Dr C. N. Griffin.

THE GENITAL TRACT

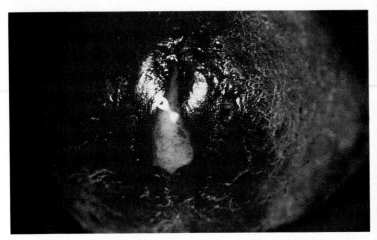

Fig. 78 Gonococcal urethritis. Typical purulent meatal discharge with inflammation of the glans. Symptomatic gonorrhoea in males is characterized by a spontaneous purulent discharge and dysuria. Courtesy of Dr J. Clay.

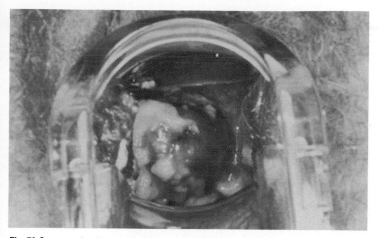

Fig. 79 Gonococcal endocervicitis. View through vaginal speculum showing reddened external os through which mucopurulent secretion is exuding. The most common manifestation of gonorrhoea in females is cervicitis, which is often asymptomatic. Courtesy of Dr S. E. Thompson.

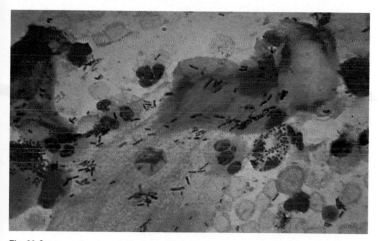

Fig. 80 Gonococcal endocervicitis. Gram stain of pus from cervix. This illustrates the difficulty which may be experienced in identifying *Neisseria gonorrhoeae* microscopically in infected females, since its presence is often obscured by other bacteria. Courtesy of Dr S. E. Thompson.

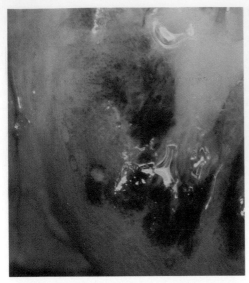

Fig. 81 Chlamydia endocervicitis. Colposcopic view showing mucopurulent discharge and beefy red mucosa of columnar epithelium. This lesion, which is usually asymptomatic, should be looked for in sexual partners of men with non-gonococcal urethritis. Courtesy of Mr D. W. Sturdee.

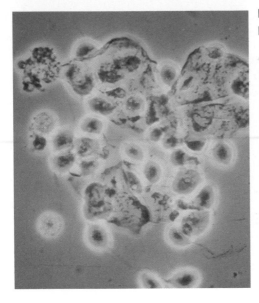

Fig. 82 Trichomoniasis. Wet preparation of *Trichomonas vaginalis*. Direct examination of vaginal secretion shows pus cells interspersed with the pear-shaped, nucleated and flagellated protozoan organisms. Vaginitis due to *T. vaginalis* results in a profuse, thin, frothy, offensive discharge. Most infections in males are asymptomatic. Simultaneous treatment of all sexual partners is necessary to prevent reinfection. Courtesy of Dr S. E. Thompson.

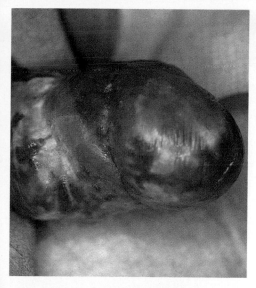

Fig. 83 Candida balanitis. Intensely pruritic inflammation of the glans and prepuce with white cheesy exudate. This lesion is usually seen in sexual partners of women with vaginal candidiasis. Courtesy of Dr J. Clay.

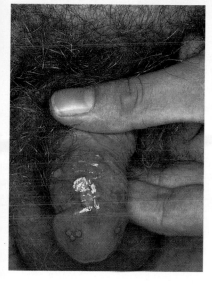

Fig. 84 Genital herpes. Primary infection of the penis showing groups of typical painful ulcers on the glans and shaft. The ulcers result from rupture of the initial vesicular lesions. Courtesy of Dr B. K. Fisher.

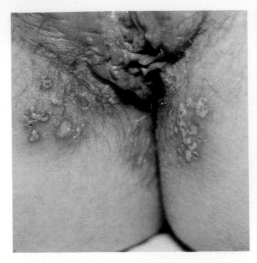

Fig. 85 Genital herpes. Vesicles and ulcers on the labia and surrounding skin. The virus can be visualized by electron microscopy, or cultured from the vesicular fluid. Courtesy of Dr J. Clay.

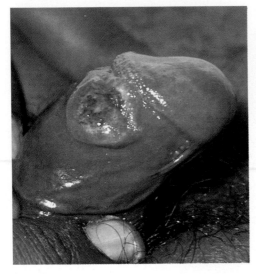

Fig. 86 Primary syphilis. Typical penile chancre showing rounded, raised and well-defined lesion with central ulceration. The lesion and the enlarged lymph nodes are both painless. Courtesy of Dr R. D. Catterall.

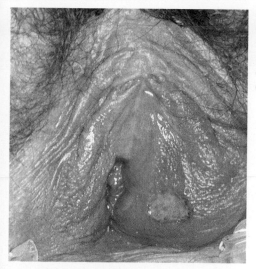

Fig. 87 Primary syphilis. A well-defined chancre on the labia minora. The base of the ulcer is clear with a shallow covering of slough. Courtesy of Dr R. D. Catterall.

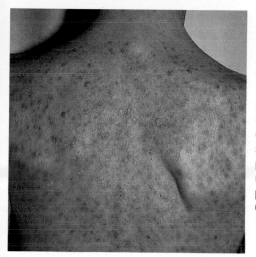

Fig. 88 Papular syphilide of secondary syphilis. The papules are widely distributed. Each lesion is rounded, discrete and slightly indurated. Involvement of the palms and soles is characteristic and aids in the diagnosis. The rash of secondary syphilis is often papular, as seen here, but may also be macular, psoriasiform or pustular. Courtesy of Dr B. K. Fisher.

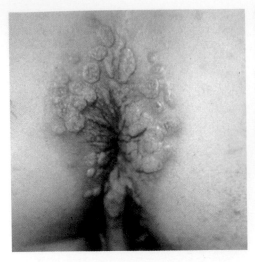

Fig. 89 Secondary syphilis. Condylomata of the perianal area. Large papular lesions with well-defined margins and pale irregular surfaces which tend to ulcerate. These lesions are swarming with spirochaetes and are highly infectious. Courtesy of Dr R. D. Catterall.

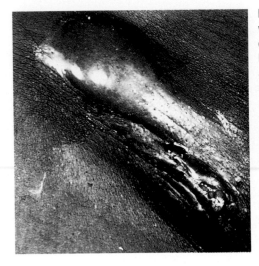

Fig. 90 Lymphogranuloma venereum. The bubo of chronic inguinal lymphadenopathy. The nodes are matted together by inflammatory periadenitis and a sinus is also visible. This disease, caused by certain serovars of *Chlamydia trachomatis*, is seen primarily in subtropical and tropical countries. In females and homosexual males painful proctitis and suppuration of perirectal glands may occur and lead to chronic rectal strictures and fistulae. Courtesy of Dr S. Olansky.

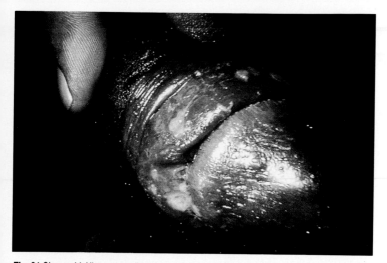

Fig. 91 Chancroid. Ulcers extending along the coronal sulcus of the penis. They are irregular in shape, painful and not indurated, all points of distinction from syphilitic chancre. Chancroid occurs primarily in developing countries but is occasionally found among the poorest individuals living in certain large cities in industrialized countries. Courtesy of Dr S. Olansky.

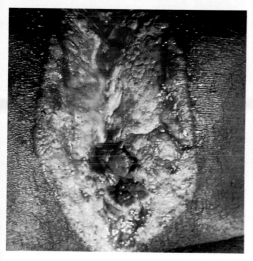

Fig. 92 Granuloma inguinale. A large area of ulceration in the perianal area with a friable, irregular granulomatous base. Some areas have bled and scabbed. This chronic, progressive destructive infection is seen mainly in tropical and subtropical countries and is rare in the West. Courtesy of Dr T. F. Sellers, Jr.

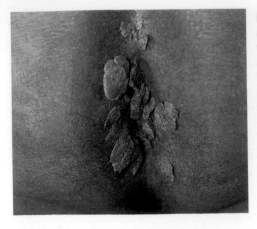

Fig. 93 Condylomata acuminata. Several large fleshy lesions around the anus of a homosexual male. It is important to examine the anal canal and lower rectum to determine the precise extent of the problem. Courtesy of Dr L. Parish.

BONES AND JOINTS

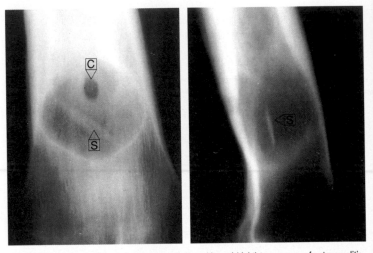

Fig. 94 Acute osteomyelitis. Anteroposterior (left) and lateral (right) tomograms of osteomyelitis of the femur showing an area of bone destruction containing sequestrum (S). There is a hole in the bone (cloaca – arrow C) posteriorly, where the infection has broken through the cortex to form a sinus tract. Courtesy of Dr D. C. Tudway.

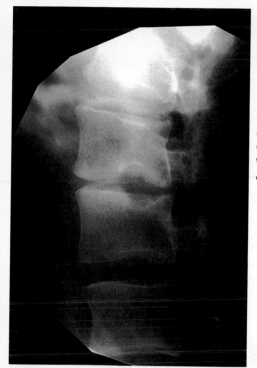

Fig. 95 Vertebral osteomyelitis. Lateral radiograph of the lumbar spine (top), and lateral (centre) and anteroposterior (bottom) CT scan reconstructions, showing narrowing of the disk space and early destruction of the end-plates of two adjacent vertebrae. Courtesy of Mr R. J. Cherry.

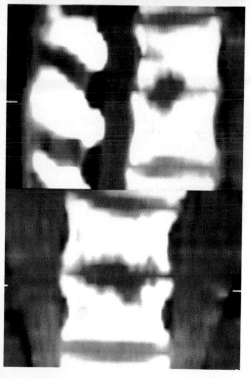

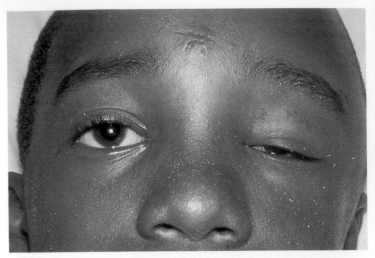

Fig. 96 Acute osteomyelitis. Osteomyelitis of the right frontal bone due to *Staphylococcus aureus*, secondary to infection in the right frontal sinus ('Pott's puffy tumour'). Courtesy of Dr T. F. Sellers, Jr.

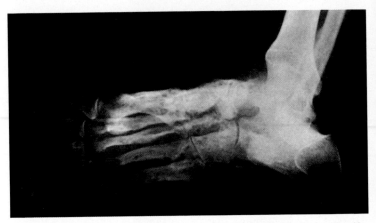

Fig. 97 Madura foot. This is a chronic, progressive, localized destructive infection involving skin, subcutaneous tissues, muscle and bone. It is caused by soil organisms, including a number of different species of fungi. The granulomatous process gradually destroys the architecture of the involved bones and soft tissues, with production of deep abscesses and multiple draining fistulous tracts.

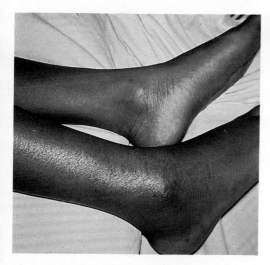

Fig. 98 Gonococcal septic arthritis. Arthritis due to *Neisseria gonorrhoeae* in a 24-year-old woman showing marked erythema and swelling of the right ankle and leg. By courtesy of Dr T. F. Sellers, Jr.

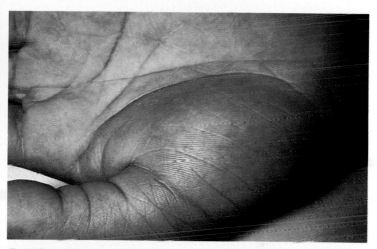

Fig. 99 Gonococcal tenosynovitis of the left thumb secondary to gonococcal bacteraemia. Note the erythema and swelling of the thenar eminence. Tenosynovitis is a relatively common manifestation of gonococcal bacteraemia, and may provide a clue to the aetiological diagnosis. Courtesy of Dr T. F. Sellers, Jr.

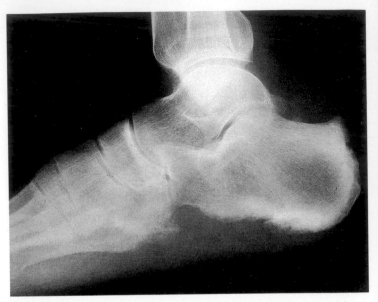

Fig. 100 Reiter's syndrome. Radiograph of foot showing calcaneal spurs with characteristic 'fluffy' appearance. The posterior and inferior surfaces of the os calcis are affected. Heel pain is a fairly common manifestation of this disease. Courtesy of Dr S. Olansky.

THE CARDIOVASCULAR SYSTEM

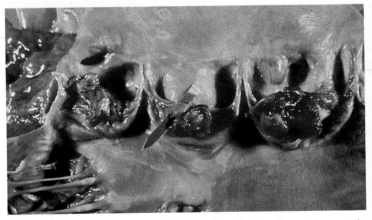

Fig. 101 Bacterial endocarditis. Endocarditis involving the aortic valve with vegetations on each of the three cusps and perforation of the non-coronary cusp.

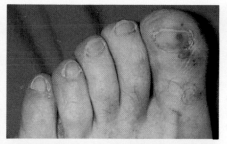

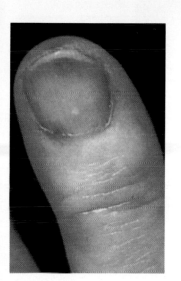

Fig. 102 Bacterial endocarditis. Widespread skin lesions may sometimes be seen, especially in acute staphylococcal endocarditis. The patient showed numerous ecchymoses of his hands and feet during the course of staphylococcal septicaemia, and signs of aortic valve involvement soon appeared.

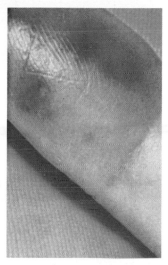

Fig. 103 Two diagnostically important manifestations of infective endocarditis are splinter haemorrhages (left) and Osler's nodes (right). These painful erythematous nodular lesions may be due to deposition of immune complexes in blood vessel walls, but bacteria have been cultured from them in a few instances, suggesting that they may be embolic in nature. Courtesy of Dr J. F. John, Jr.

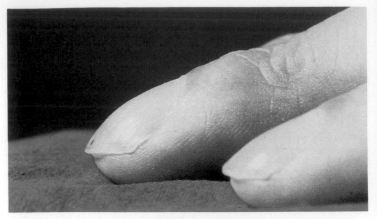

Fig. 104 Bacterial endocarditis. Clubbing of the fingers in long-standing subacute bacterial endocarditis.

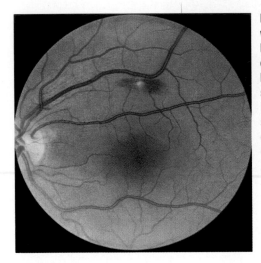

Fig. 105 Roth spot. This white-centred retinal haemorrhage is an important diagnostic sign of bacteraemia, most commonly seen in bacterial endocarditis. It is however occasionally seen in non-infectious conditions such as systemic erythematosus and leukaemia.

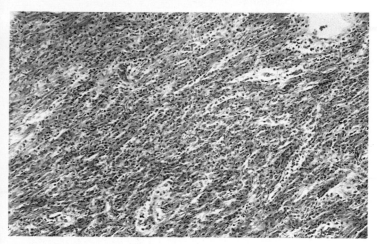

Fig. 106 Acute Coxsackie B myocarditis. Inflammatory cell infiltrate, widening of the interstitium and some hypertrophy and malalignment of the myocardial fibres. Mumps, influenza and Epstein-Barr viruses may cause a similar lesion. There is often an associated pericarditis. Courtesy of Dr C. Edwards.

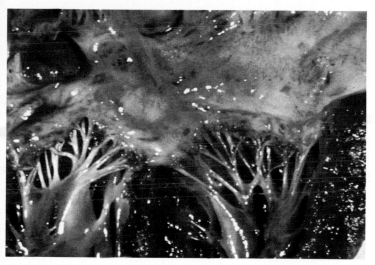

Fig. 107 Acute rheumatic fever. Mitral valvulitis showing thickening of chordae tendineae and valve leaflets, with small verrucae along the line of valve closure.

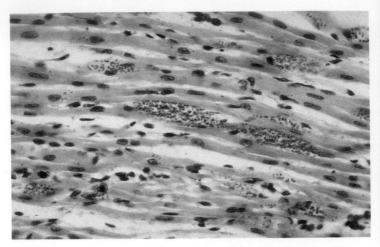

Fig. 108 Chagas' disease. Myocarditis showing amastigote forms of *Trypanosoma cruzi* in cardiac muscle. (H&E stain.) This is from a case of acute infection. In chronic Chagas' disease myocarditis organisms are scarce, and there is loss of parasympathetic neurons and muscle fibres with chronic inflammation and fibrosis.

SKIN AND SOFT TISSUE
Bacterial, protozoal and helminth infections

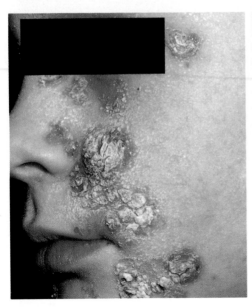

Fig. 109 Impetigo. This is a highly communicable superficial infection of the skin, caused by *Streptococcus pyogenes* or *Staphylococcus aureus*, almost exclusively affecting young children in warm climates. The characteristic yellow crusts are often the main feature on presentation.

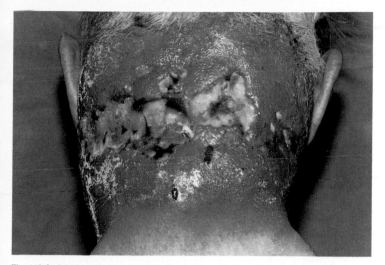

Fig. 110 Carbuncle. A huge area of induration of the neck with multiple discharging follicular abscesses. This condition, which begins as a furuncle (boil), is almost always caused by *Staphylococcus aureus*. The infection extends through the skin into the subcutaneous fat and may extend over a large area, usually on the nape of the neck or back. Surgical drainage as well as treatment with antistaphylococcal antibiotics is required for effective treatment.

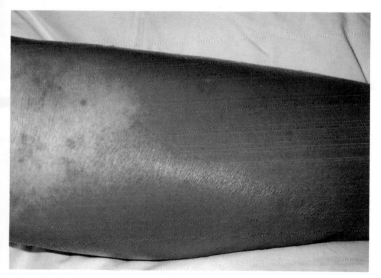

Fig. 111 Cellulitis. Erythematous area with ill-defined margin over lower limb. This is a spreading superficial infection of the skin, usually caused by group A β-haemolytic streptococci or *Staphylococcus aureus*, or both.

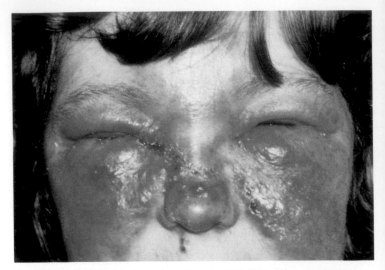

Fig. 112 Erysipelas. A typical butterfly-wing rash on the checks. Both eyes are closed by oedema of the lids. This form of cellulitis is almost always caused by *Streptococcus pyogenes*. The lesions are bright red, shiny and painful, with a sharply demarcated edge. It is most common on the legs or face and is often symmetrically distributed. The oedema and induration are caused by invasion and obstruction of the lymphatics in the skin.

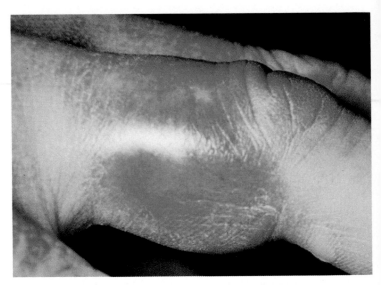

Fig. 113 Erysipeloid. Characteristic indolent, purple, non-purulent swelling of the finger, one of the most common sites of infection. Erysipeloid is an occupational disease of people handling fish and meat. The causative organism, *Erysipelothrix rhusiopathiae*, is a gram-positive rod found in many wild and domestic mammals, fish and fowl.

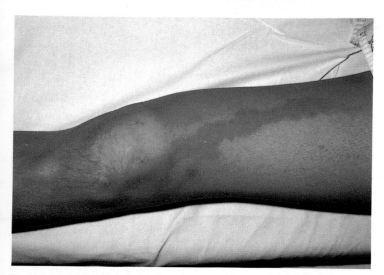

Fig. 114 Lymphangitis. Inflamed lymphatic channels extending up the thigh to regional lymph nodes from an area of cellulitis of the lower leg. Lymphangitis is usually a complication of group A streptococcal infection of the skin of a limb and is often accompanied by tender regional lymphadenopathy, fever and occasionally bacteraemia.

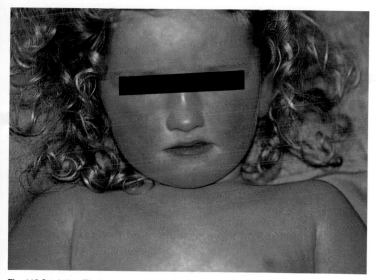

Fig. 115 Scarlatina. The face appears flushed with circumoral pallor. Scarlet fever is due to group A β-haemolytic streptococci which produce an erythrogenic toxin. The rash blanches upon pressure, and may impart a sandpaper-like texture to the skin. The erythema often spares the area around the mouth but is accentuated in the creases of the elbow, groin and axillary folds (Pastia's lines). Other features are 'strawberry tongue' (see Fig. 6) and eventual desquamation of the tongue and skin.

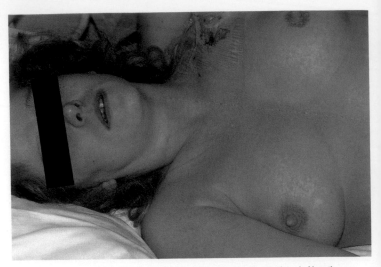

Fig. 116 Toxic shock syndrome. Typical sunburn-like rash over face and trunk. Note the dryness and hyperaemia of the lips. Other features of this syndrome are fever, hypotension, involvement of multiple organ systems and eventual desquamation of the skin. Most cases are due to a toxin produced by *Staphylococcus aureus*, but a few cases have been reported in association with infections due to *Streptococcus pyogenes*.

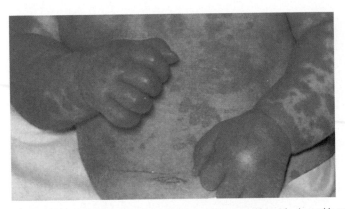

Fig. 117 Kawasaki disease. Red indurated oedema of the extremities and polymorphic rash in a child with Kawasaki disease (mucocutaneous lymph node syndrome). The aetiology of this condition is unknown but it is presumed to be an infection. Other features are persistent fever, dry, red, oral mucous membranes and conjunctival congestion. Treatment with intravenous γ-globulin is effective.

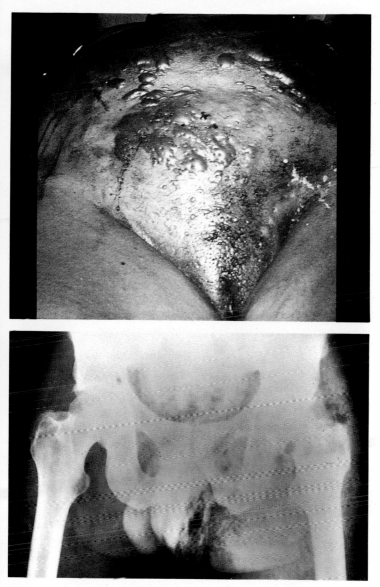

Fig. 118 Necrotizing fasciitis of the abdominal wall. Top: Multiple bullae and blackened areas of skin. Bottom: A soft tissue radiograph of the same patient shows gas in the tissues. This severe infection of the subcutaneous tissues and superficial fascia arises as a result of trauma or surgery in the presence of faecal soiling, or spreads from a perirectal abscess. The bacterial aetiology is a mixture of peptostreptococci, *Bacteroides* species and facultative anaerobes such as Enterobacteriaceae and streptococci. Effective treatment requires extensive surgical debridement as well as antibiotics active against the causative microorganisms. Courtesy of Dr W. M. Rambo.

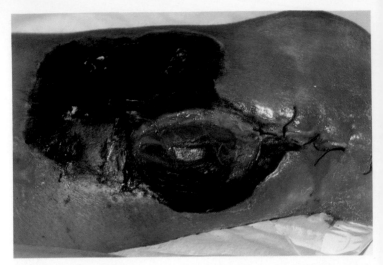

Fig. 119 Gas gangrene. There is a serosanguinous discharge from the lower end of the surgical wound and the affected muscles show pallor and failure to bleed. Gas gangrene (clostridial myonecrosis) is a fulminant life-threatening infection of skeletal muscle caused by toxins of *Clostridium perfringens*. Immediate and extensive surgical debridement, gas gangrene antitoxin, antibiotics and hyperbaric oxygen constitute optimum treatment.

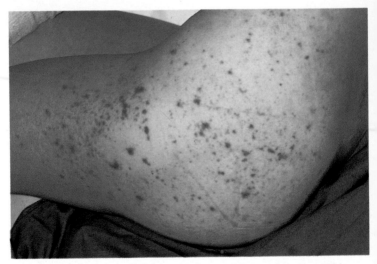

Fig. 120 Acute meningococcaemia. Purpuric lesions of variable size on buttocks and thighs. The rash of meningococcaemia is at first macular, then petechial and purpuric, sometimes with ecchymoses of up to several centimetres in diameter with an irregular edge. Gram-negative diplococci can occasionally be seen on smears obtained from these lesions.

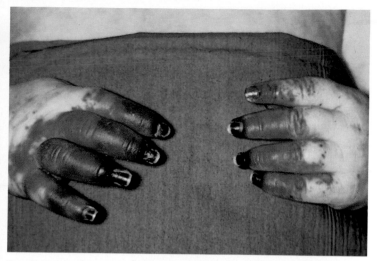

Fig. 121 Acute meningococcaemia. Gangrene of the extremities following a near-fatal illness with hypotension.

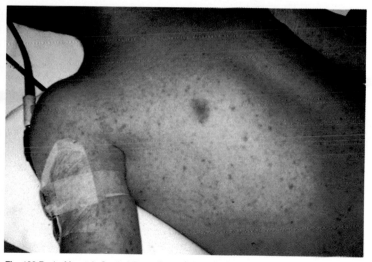

Fig. 122 Rocky Mountain Spotted Fever. Seventh day of illness in a young boy. A moderately severe eruption with macular and petechial elements of various sizes. The rash usually appears after several days of fever and is absent in about 10% of cases. It starts peripherally and spreads centrally to the trunk. It is initially macular but later becomes petechial and purpuric. It often involves the palms and soles, and lesions may sometimes be seen within the oral cavity. Courtesy of Dr T. F. Sellers, Jr.

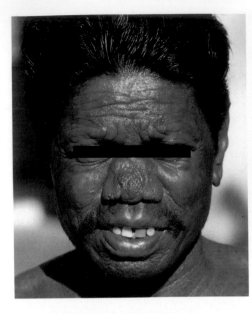

Fig. 123 Lepromatous leprosy. Typical 'leonine' facies with thickened infiltrated skin, widened nose and loss of eyebrows. The thickening of the skin is due to infiltration of the dermis with enormous numbers of the causative acid-fast bacillus, *Mycobacterium leprae.* Courtesy of Dr D. A. Lewis.

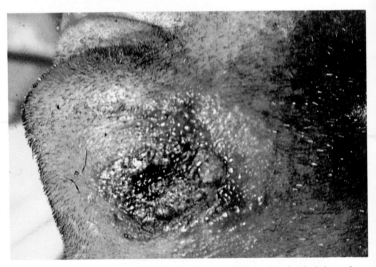

Fig. 124 Anthrax. The characteristic black eschar is surrounded by a ring of vesiculation and a wide area of non-pitting gelatinous oedema. Fluid from the vesicles or from beneath the eschar shows large gram-positive bacilli (*Bacillus anthracis*), often in chains. Courtesy of Dr F. J. Nye.

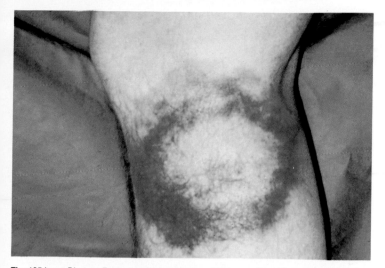

Fig. 125 Lyme Disease. Rash of erythema chronicum migrans on leg surrounding the site of a tick bite. This characteristic lesion is present in approximately 60% of cases. The disease, caused by the spirochaete *Borrelia burgdorferi*, is transmitted by ticks, primarily *Ixodes dammini*. In the later stages musculoskeletal, cardiac and neurological manifestations may appear. Courtesy of Dr E. Sahn.

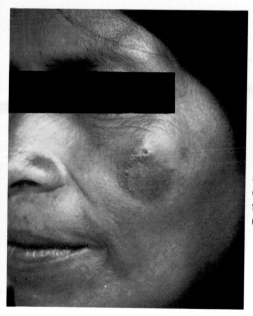

Fig. 126 American leishmaniasis. Early lesion caused by *Leishmania braziliensis* on the face of a young woman. Leishmaniasis is a complex of diverse diseases caused by protozoan organisms of the genus *Leishmania*, species of which are found in both the Old World and the New World. It is a zoonosis affecting rodents, dogs and other mammals, transmitted by sandflies. Courtesy of Dr P. J. Cooper.

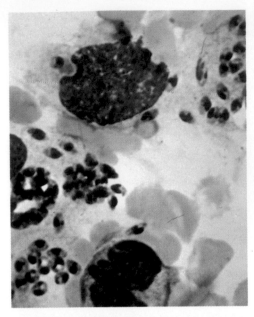

Fig. 127 American leishmaniasis. Leishmanial organisms within macrophages in aspirate from a lesion of leishmaniasis.

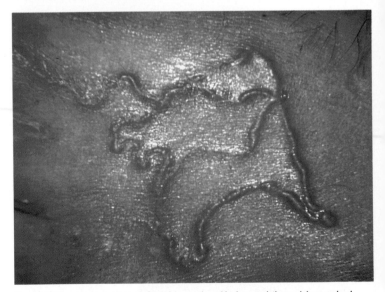

Fig. 128 Cutaneous larva migrans. Creeping eruption with characteristic serpiginous raised lesion. The lesions develop as a result of infection with larval nematodes of various species, usually dog or cat hookworms of low human pathogenicity. The track marks the route of the parasite as it burrows through the skin. Courtesy of Dr K. A. Riley.

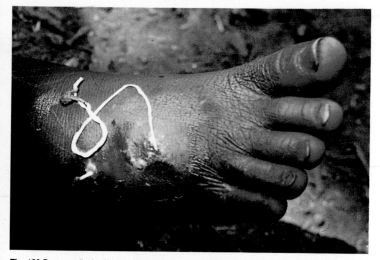

Fig. 129 Dracunculiasis. Adult female Guinea worm (*Dracunculus medinensis*) emerging from the foot of a young child. The foot is swollen and there is cellulitis due to secondary bacterial infection along the track of the worm. The infection is acquired by ingesting water containing infected crustaceans (copepods), primarily of the genus *Cyclops*. After treatment with an appropriate anti-helminthic agent, the adult worm can be removed by gently rolling it around a small stick.

SKIN AND SOFT TISSUE
Viral, fungal and ectoparasitic infections

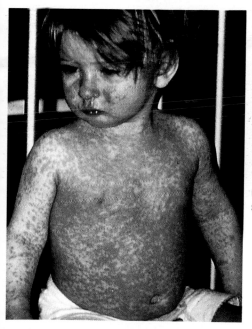

Fig. 130 Measles. This is a very characteristic picture. A miserable child, with a blotchy rash, runny nose and bleary eyes. The rash is denser on the face than on the trunk and has a purple tinge. In fair-skinned patients after the severe illness has subsided there is much 'staining' of the areas affected by the rash. This purpuric rash lasts a few more days but leaves no sequelae.

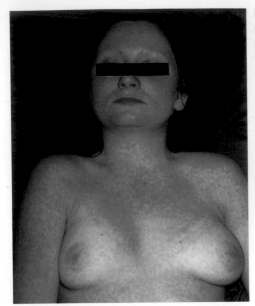

Fig. 131 Rubella. The rash of rubella consists of discrete pink macules, although the facial eruption is often confluent. The face and trunk are affected most on the first day and the rash then spreads downwards and peripherally. Generalized lymphadenopathy precedes and accompanies the rash. The features of rubella vary greatly and clinical diagnosis is unreliable.

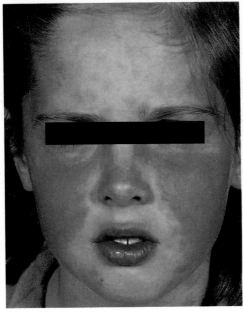

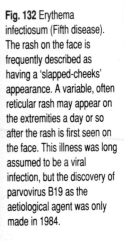

Fig. 132 Erythema infectiosum (Fifth disease). The rash on the face is frequently described as having a 'slapped-cheeks' appearance. A variable, often reticular rash may appear on the extremities a day or so after the rash is first seen on the face. This illness was long assumed to be a viral infection, but the discovery of parvovirus B19 as the aetiological agent was only made in 1984.

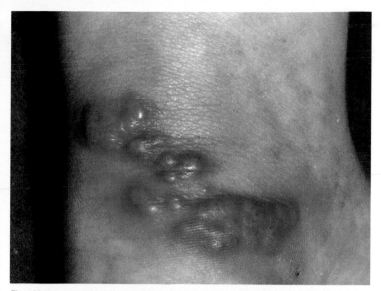

Fig. 133 Herpes simplex. Primary infection on the wrist of a young man, acquired through judo. Primary infections with HSV may occur on the skin as a result of direct inoculation during wrestling (herpes gladiatorum) or other contact sports. Infections of the finger (herpetic whitlows) often occur in dental technicians or in nurses working in intensive care units.

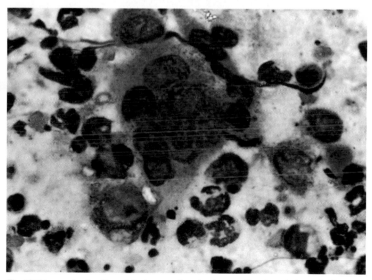

Fig. 134 Herpes simplex. Tzanck test preparation showing a multinucleated giant cell. (Wright's stain.) This technique does not distinguish HSV infection from infections due to varicella–zoster virus. This distinction can be made using monoclonal antibody tests or viral culture. Courtesy of Dr H. P. Holley, Jr.

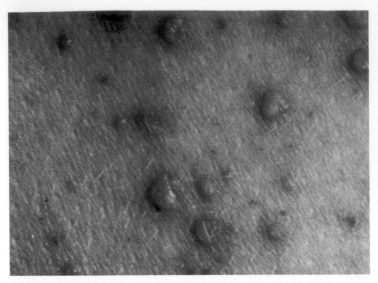

Fig. 135 Varicella (Chickenpox). Early rash showing lesions at various stages: macules, papules and superficial vesicles, some beginning to inspissate.

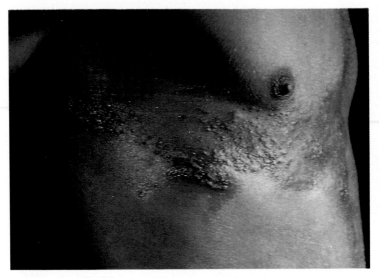

Fig. 136 Herpes zoster. Lesions in a dermatomal distribution on the thorax. Although most lesions heal uneventfully, scarring in the affected areas is not uncommon and the scars may become keloidal. Courtesy of Dr J. F. John, Jr.

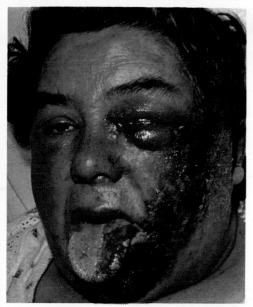

Fig. 137 Herpes zoster. Lesions in the distribution of the mandibular division of the trigeminal nerve. Courtesy of Dr G. D. W. McKendrick.

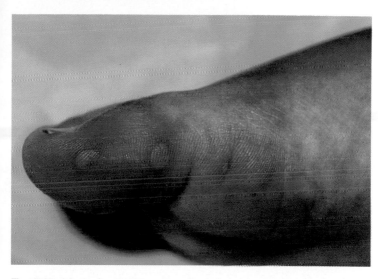

Fig. 138 Hand, foot and mouth disease. Several vesicular lesions on the foot. This disease, caused by Coxsackie virus A16 (occasionally by A5 or A10), usually occurs in children under the age of ten years. Vesicular lesions are also seen in the oral cavity, and there may also be a macular or petechial rash on the buttocks and thighs.

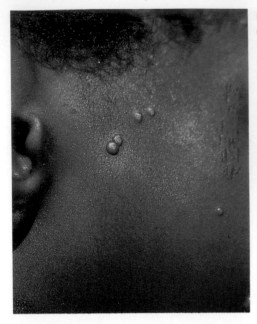

Fig. 139 Molluscum contagiosum. Several fleshy lesions with umbilicated centres on the face. The lesions, caused by an unclassified member of the poxvirus family, tend to regress and disappear within a few months except in patients with AIDS, in whom they may continue to spread and enlarge.

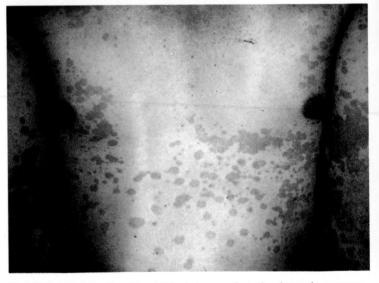

Fig. 140 Tinea versicolor. Brownish-red diffuse lesions over the trunk and arms of a young man. This superficial dermatomycosis is caused by the lipophilic yeast, *Malassezia furfur*. Courtesy of Dr E. Sahn.

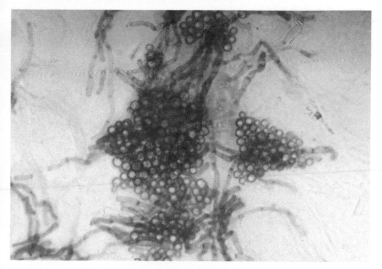

Fig. 141 Tinea versicolor. Sticky tape strip showing typical cluster of round budding cells and mycelial elements ('spaghetti and meatballs') of *Malassezia furfur*. Methylene blue stain. Courtesy of Ms A. E. Prevost.

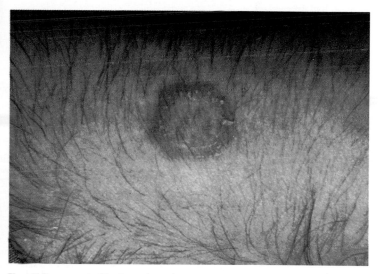

Fig. 142 Tinea corporis. Classic annular erythematous lesion ('ringworm') due to *Microsporum* species showing an advancing active periphery and scaling in the central area. Courtesy of Ms A. E. Prevost.

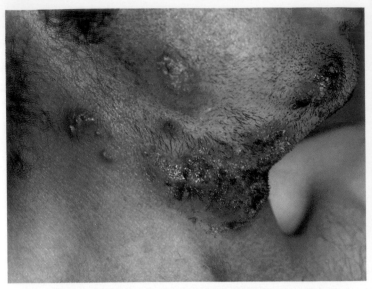

Fig. 143 Tinea barbae (barber's itch). Chronic dermatomycosis of the beard area of the face and neck with both superficial lesions and deeper lesions involving the hair follicles.

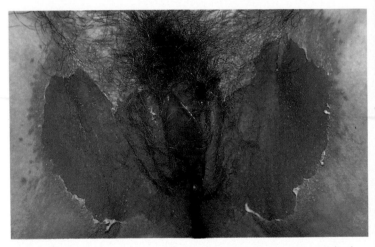

Fig. 144 Candidiasis of the external genitalia and perineum. The vulva and labia are red and intensely pruritic, and there are large areas of denuded skin with well-defined edges and some scaling. Satellite lesions are visible beyond the edges. This is often associated with vaginal candidiasis.

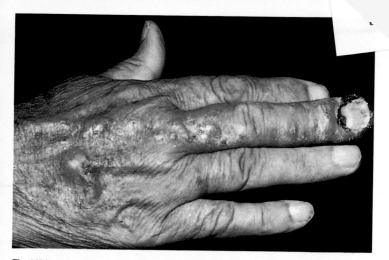

Fig. 145 Lymphocutaneous sporotrichosis. A chronic crusting primary lesion involving the nail bed of the third finger, with multiple painless nodules along the lymphatic channels draining this lesion. This infection, caused by the saprophytic fungus *Sporothrix schenckii*, is seen most commonly in plant nurserymen, rose gardeners and others who handle sphagnum moss. Granuloma formation and microabscesses are seen on histopathological examination. Courtesy of Dr T. F. Sellers, Jr.

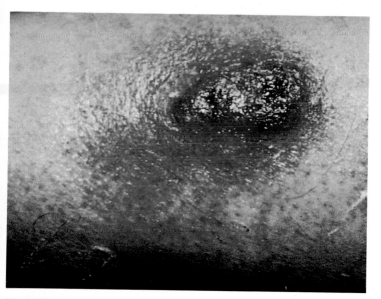

Fig. 146 Blastomycosis. Typical raised, crusting, proliferative cutaneous lesion in a patient with chronic blastomycosis. The lung is the usual portal of entry for the dimorphic fungus *Blastomyces dermatiditis*; the skin lesions result from haematogenous dissemination. Courtesy of Dr K. A. Riley.

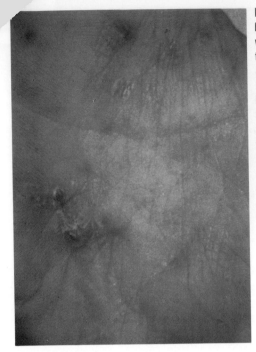

Fig. 147 Scabies. Minute burrows can be seen together with papules. Scabies is due to infestation by the mite *Sarcoptes scabiei* var. *hominis*, the female of which burrows into the skin of the host, laying its eggs in the base of the stratum corneum of the epidermis. Diagnosis is made by the appearance of the intensely pruritic lesions, or by scraping the burrow with a scalpel blade covered with mineral oil and finding the mites and eggs on microscopic examination.

THE EYE

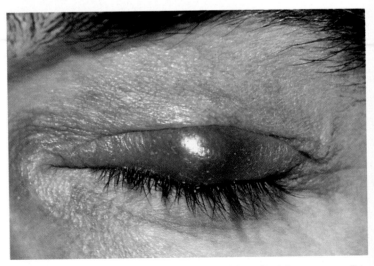

Fig. 148 Acute stye. Acute inflammation of the upper eyelid due to *Staphylococcus aureus*. This infection of the glands of the eyelash follicle presents as a localized painful abscess on the lid margin. Courtesy of Dr A. N. Carlson.

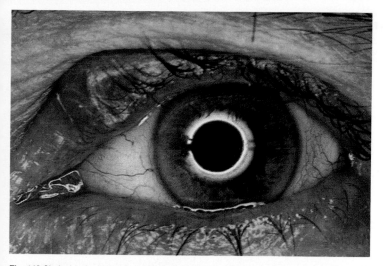

Fig. 149 Chalazion. Local redness and swelling due to granulomatous inflammation of the Meibomian gland, usually caused by *Staphylococcus aureus*. Courtesy of Mr R. J. Marsh.

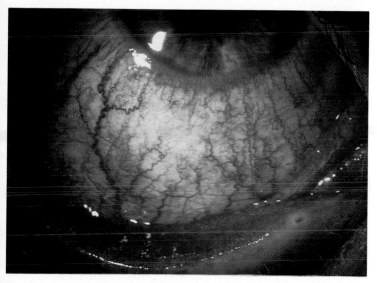

Fig. 150 Acute conjunctivitis. Typical distribution of hyperaemia, diminishing in severity towards the cornea. In iritis, the hyperaemia is greatest at the limbus. Acute conjunctivitis may be caused by a number of different viruses, bacteria and *Chlamydia* species. Courtesy of Mr S. Harding.

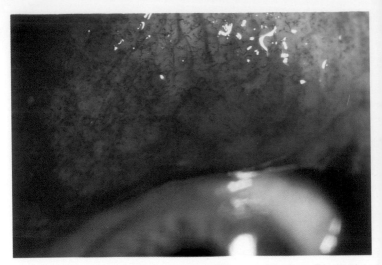

Fig. 151 TRIC conjunctivitis. A typical case with large follicles in the lower fornix. This type of follicular conjunctivitis occurs in neonates or sexually active adults and is caused by subgroups D–K of *Chlamydia trachomatis*. The source of the organisms is the genital tract of both women and men. By courtesy of Mr P. A. Hunter.

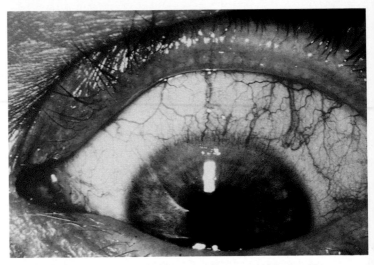

Fig. 152 Trachoma. Early involvement of the cornea with new vessel formation at the upper margin. Trachoma is a chronic follicular conjunctivitis caused by serogroups A–C of *Chlamydia trachomatis*. Untreated it may result in severe scarring of the conjunctiva and cornea and is a major cause of blindness in areas of the world with poor standards of hygiene. Courtesy of Mr G. Gatford.

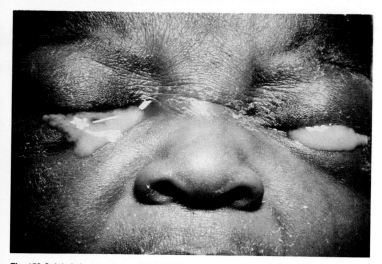

Fig. 153 Ophthalmia neonatorum. Marked bilateral purulent discharge in a neonate, caused by *Staphylococcus aureus*. The disease results from contamination of the neonate's eye during birth; the most common aetiological agents are *Chlamydia trachomatis, Neisseria gonorrhoeae* and *Staphylococcus aureus*. By courtesy of Dr P. Dobson.

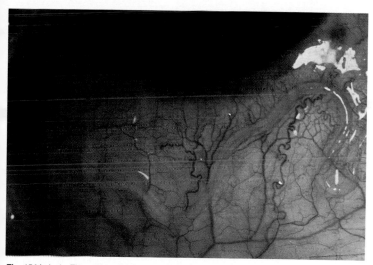

Fig. 154 Loiasis. Threadlike adult *Loa loa* migrating in the subconjunctival tissues. This filarial nematode is endemic in West and Central Africa. The larval form is transmitted from human to human by the diurnally-biting banana fly (genus *Chrysops*). The larvae develop into adult worms, which migrate through the subcutaneous tissues and sometimes beneath the conjunctiva. Courtesy of Teaching Aids at Low Cost, Institute of Child Health, London.

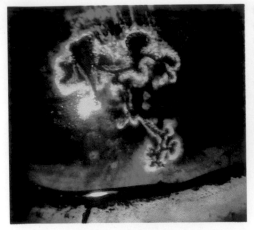

Fig. 155 Herpes simplex. A dendritic ulcer. (Fluorescein stain.) HSV is the most important viral cause of keratitis. The ulcerative lesions may be extremely chronic and lead to scarring and vascularization. Topical therapy with acyclovir, trifluridine or other antiviral agents may be effective.

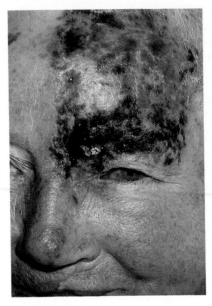

Fig. 156 Herpes zoster ophthalmicus. Involvement of the nasociliary branch of the trigeminal nerve produces vesicles on the tip of the nose and is generally associated with corneal involvement. Courtesy of Mr S. Harding.

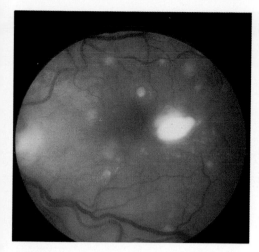

Fig. 157 Candida endophthalmitis. Fundus photograph showing patches of white fluffy exudate. These may be the only evidence of systemic candidiasis. It is associated with the use of intravascular catheters, immunosuppression, the use of broad-spectrum antibiotics and heroin addiction. Courtesy of Dr A. M. Geddes.

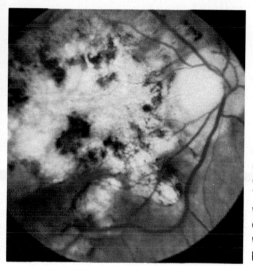

Fig. 158 Toxoplasmosis. Fundus photograph showing large areas of chorioretinitis with irregular scarring and pigmentation. Ocular toxoplasmosis is usually the result of congenital infection; infected infants may appear normal at birth but reactivation of the disease can produce chorioretinitis in later childhood or early adult life. The appearance is diagnostic, with a focal destructive chorioretinitis which leaves well-defined, heavily pigmented scars.

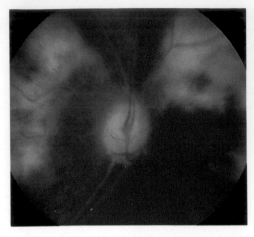

Fig. 159 Cytomegalovirus retinitis. Fundus photograph in a severe case in a patient with AIDS, showing haemorrhages and white retinal infiltration producing the 'tomato sauce and salad dressing' appearance. By courtesy of Mr D. S. I. Taylor.

SYSTEMIC INFECTIONS

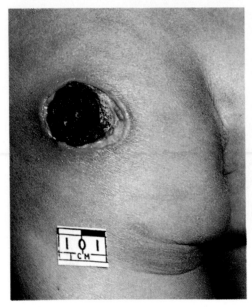

Fig. 160 Ecthyma gangrenosum. Necrotic round lesion on the buttock of a child with *Pseudomonas* septicaemia associated with immunodeficiency. This organism often multiplies in the walls of blood vessels, causing vasculitis, thrombosis and ischaemic infarction of areas of skin.

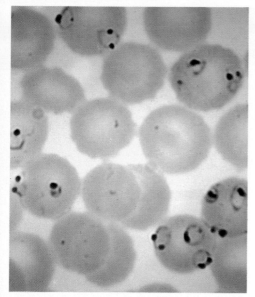

Fig. 161 Malaria. Thin blood film showing trophozoites (ring forms) of *Plasmodium falciparum*. Note two parasites within the same red cell and double chromatin knobs. Giemsa stain. Courtesy of Dr D. Lewis.

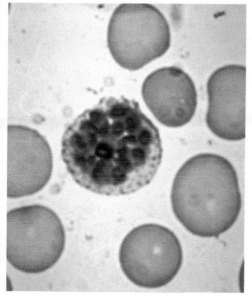

Fig. 162 Malaria. Thin blood film showing fully-developed schizont of *Plasmodium vivax* with merozoites ready to burst out. Giemsa stain. Courtesy of Dr D. Lewis.

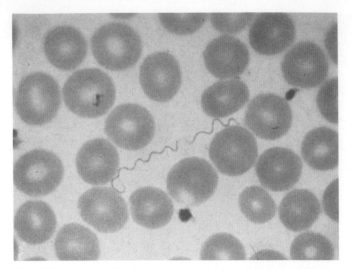

Fig. 163 Relapsing fever. This picture may be seen in either epidemic louse-borne human disease caused by *Borrelia recurrentis* or the tick-borne zoonosis caused by various *Borrelia* species. During the febrile phase the organisms are present in the blood either as tightly-coiled helical spirochaetes as shown here, or as loosely-coiled forms. Courtesy of Dr T. F. Sellers, Jr.

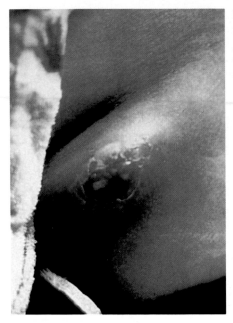

Fig. 164 Plague. In bubonic plague, the most common form of *Yersinia pestis* infection in humans, the organisms multiply rapidly at the site of the bite of an infected flea and spread to the regional lymph nodes, producing the characteristic suppurative lymphadenitis (bubo). This patient exhibits an advanced stage of inguinal lymphadenitis in which the lymph nodes have undergone suppuration and the lesion has drained spontaneously. Courtesy of Dr J. R. Cantey.

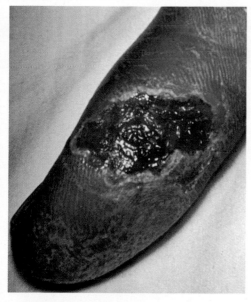

Fig. 165 Tularaemia. Irregular ulcer at the site of the initial lesion. In the common ulceroglandular form of tularaemia, caused by *Francisella tularensis*, there is an infected nodule at the site of inoculation which later ulcerates, with local lymph node enlargement. Courtesy of Dr T. F. Sellers, Jr.

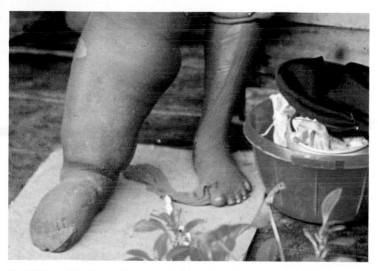

Fig. 166 Bancroftian filariasis. Pronounced oedema of the right leg in a woman in Puerto Limon, Costa Rica. Presence of adult filarial worms in the lymphatic vessels results in chronic lymphangitis and lymphadenitis with progressive lymphoedema. Courtesy of Dr R. Muller.

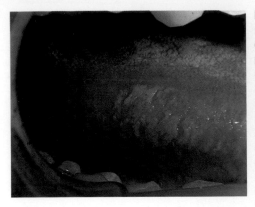

Fig. 167 Hairy leukoplakia. Raised white lesions of the oral mucosa, usually most prominent along the lateral aspect of the tongue. It is seen almost exclusively in individuals with HIV infection. It is usually asymptomatic and, unlike the lesions of oral candidiasis, cannot be scraped off and does not respond to antifungal treatment. It is related to the replication of Epstein–Barr virus in keratinized cells of the tongue and buccal mucosa. Courtesy of Dr H. P. Holley.

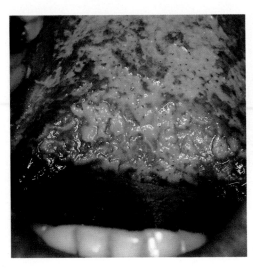

Fig. 168 Candidiasis. Extensive oral candidiasis (thrush) involving the palate. The whitish patches may be scraped off to reveal an erythematous base in individuals who are severely immunosuppressed. Candida oesophagitis is often also present.

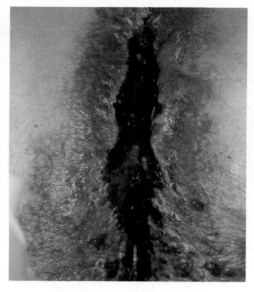

Fig. 169 Herpes simplex virus type 2 infection. Progressive, deeply eroding perianal lesion in a homosexual man with AIDS. Infection with HSV-2 occurs in more than 90% of homosexual men with HIV infection, and is usually manifested by lesions in the genital and perianal areas. These are often chronic and progressive and produce much local tissue destruction. Although the lesions respond to treatment with acyclovir, recurrence is common after treatment is discontinued and resistant variants of the virus may appear. Courtesy of Dr E. Sahn.

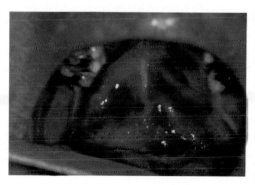

Fig. 170 Kaposi's sarcoma. Raised, dark-red lesions on the hard palate. Kaposi's sarcoma is common in individuals with advanced HIV infection, and often runs an aggressive course with extensive lesions on the skin and oral mucosa and in visceral organs. It is disproportionately common in homosexual men and heterosexual black Africans, and may be due to a distinct virus. By courtesy of Dr H L Ioachim.

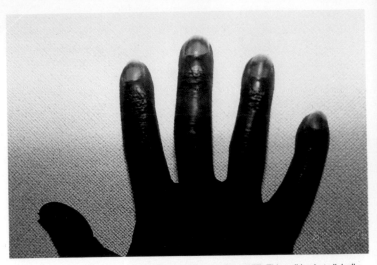

Fig. 171 Bluish discolouration of the nails in a patient receiving AZT. This striking but clinically insignificant condition is common in patients with deeply pigmented skin. Courtesy of Dr H. P. Holley.

INDEX

Location references are caption numbers.